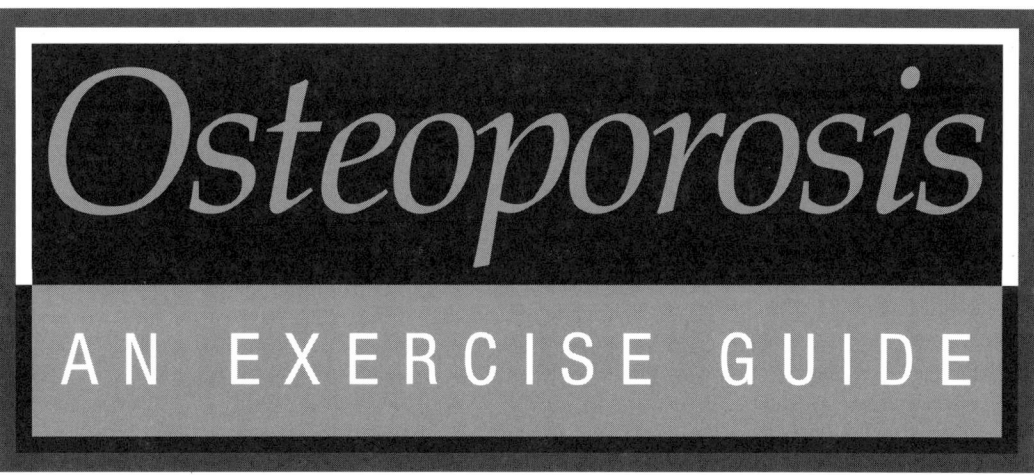

by
Margie Bissinger, MS, PT

Illustrated by Cecily Byk
Published by Workfit Consultants, L.L.C.
http://www.workfitonline.com
Design by The Barash Group
© Copyright 1998 Workfit Consultants, L.L.C., All Rights Reserved

Copying or reproducing this material is prohibited by law.

Table of Contents

Introduction 2

Exercise and Osteoporosis 3

Osteoporosis Exercise Guidelines 4

Head Forward and Up 5

Shoulder Stretch 6

Standing Back-Bend 7

Stick 'Em Up 8

Balancing on One Leg 9

Standing Side Leg Lifts 10

Standing Back Leg Lifts 11

Wall-Slide 12

Straight Leg Raise 13

All-Fours Arm and Leg Lift 14

Walking as an Exercise 15

The Walking Program 16

Heel Cord Stretch 17

Hip Flexor Stretch 18

Standing Hamstring Stretch 19

Suggested Exercise Program 20

Activities of Daily Living 21

Sitting with Support 22

Sitting without Support 23

Bending from the Hips 24

Coughing or Sneezing 25

Vacuuming, Mopping, Raking 26

Closing and References 27

Introduction

Exercise is an important step in improving your health and quality of life. As a physical therapist working with patients in the treatment and prevention of osteoporosis, I have found that people have misconceptions concerning exercise. Too often, individuals with good intentions are performing exercises that may actually cause them harm.

Many of my patients receive valuable advice on exercise from aerobic classes, home videos and fitness books. Unfortunately, these tips do not focus on the unique exercises and techniques required to provide a safe and effective program for osteoporosis prevention and treatment. That's why I developed this booklet.

Osteoporosis: An Exercise Guide is the by-product of my search for an effective, easy-to-perform program for my patients. I chose exercises that target the areas most affected by osteoporosis. By following this simple program, my patients improved their posture, strength, endurance, and balance. So can you!

There are many other safe exercises that can complement this guide. I strongly recommend consulting a physical therapist or physician before expanding this program.

Please remember, it's not the exercise that makes a successful program, it's the exerciser. Good luck on your way to building better bones!

The exercises in this book should be discussed with your physician or physical therapist prior to beginning the program.

Exercise and Osteoporosis

Osteoporosis affects more than 28 million Americans. It causes the bones to become weak and brittle. This can lead to bone fractures and other health concerns. The good news is that proper medical management, a well-designed exercise program and nutritional counseling can minimize the effects or reduce the risk of developing osteoporosis.

A complete osteoporosis exercise program should include weight-bearing, resistance, postural, and balance exercises. This booklet contains examples of all of these.

Weight-bearing exercises refer to activities where the weight of the body is transmitted through the bones, working against gravity. Your bones respond to this force by growing stronger. Walking, jogging, dancing, hiking, stair climbing and aerobic exercises are all examples of weight-bearing exercises. Bike riding and swimming, although good exercises, are not weight-bearing. Weight-bearing exercises should be performed at least three to five times per week. The goal is to work up to forty-five minutes or more per session.

Resistance exercises generate muscle tension on the bones. This strengthens the muscles and stimulates the bones to grow stronger. Exercising with weights or resistance bands are examples of this type of exercise. If you have osteoporosis, make sure to review your strength-training program in advance with your physician or physical therapist. Resistance exercises should be performed two to three times a week.

Postural exercises decrease harmful stress on the back. By performing these exercises, you can reduce your risk of spinal fractures and the rounded shoulders commonly seen with osteoporosis. These exercises should be performed throughout the day to reinforce good posture.

Balance exercises help maintain equilibrium and can reduce the risk of falling. These exercises should be performed daily.

It is important to check with your physician or physical therapist before starting any exercise program.

Osteoporosis Exercise Guidelines

- Check with your physician concerning any restrictions you may have before beginning an exercise program.

- Avoid any exercise that causes or increases pain.

- Stop exercising if you feel dizzy or short of breath.

- Never hold your breath while exercising.

- Make sure to keep your body in alignment when performing all exercises.

- Avoid exercises that involve forward bending of your spine (toe touches, sit-ups). These exercises can increase the incidence of vertebral fractures.

- Avoid exercises that involve excessive twisting (windmill toe touches). This puts too much force on your spine.

- Strive to do one set of ten repetitions of each resistance exercise. For a more challenging program, progress to three sets of ten repetitions.

- When using weights, rest one to two minutes between sets of exercises.

- When using weights, make sure to gradually increase the amount. Too much weight can be harmful.

- Wear shoes with good support and cushioning while exercising. Replace shoes when cushioning begins to wear out.

Head Forward and Up

POSTURAL EXERCISE

OBJECTIVE

To relieve tension in your neck muscles and improve posture. When the muscles in your neck are tight, your head is pulled back and down. This compresses your entire spine. To counteract this, you should perform this exercise throughout the day.

STARTING POSITION

Sit or stand in a comfortable position.

EXERCISE

Let the top of your head go forward and up. Visualize your head floating up to the ceiling like a helium balloon, as your spine gently lengthens.

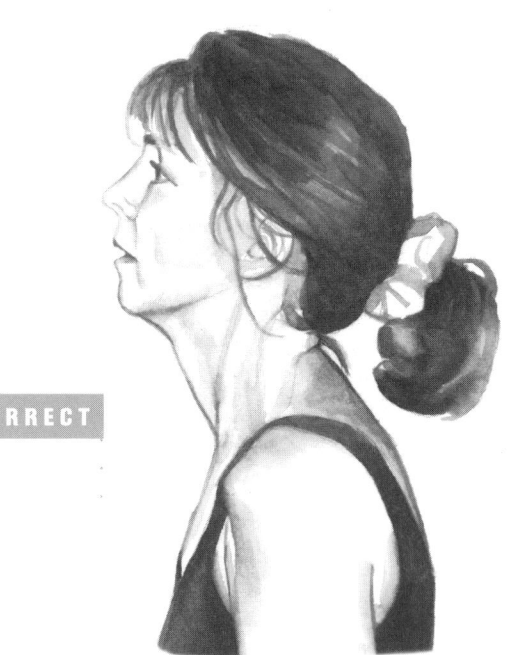

INCORRECT

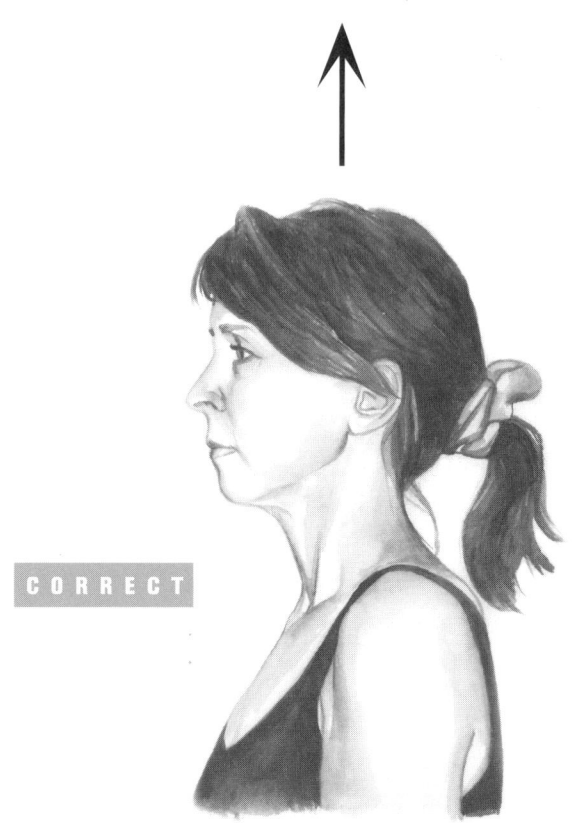

CORRECT

Shoulder Stretch

POSTURAL EXERCISE

OBJECTIVE

To improve posture and relieve tension in your neck and shoulder muscles.

When your shoulders are rounded, your upper back muscles are stretched and weakened. You can counteract this by performing this exercise three to five times per day.

STARTING POSITION

Sit at the edge of a chair.

EXERCISE

Draw your shoulders back to a comfortable position by pulling your shoulder blades together. At the same time, visualize your spine stretching up and lengthening.

Hold for three seconds.

Perform three to five repetitions.

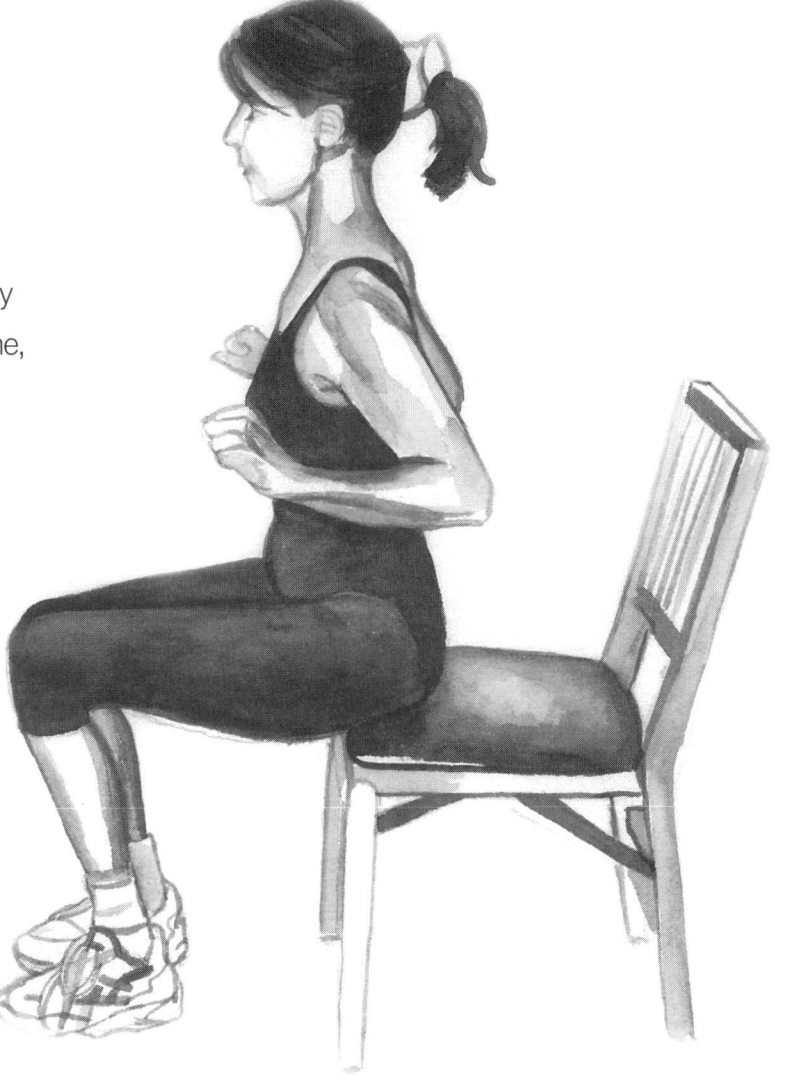

Standing Back-Bend
POSTURAL EXERCISE

OBJECTIVE

To improve posture and decrease stress on your lower back. Forward bending puts a lot of stress on your spine. Studies have indicated that forward bending exercises increase the incidence of vertebral fractures. The following exercise should be performed three to five times per day. If you have pain with backward bending, do not do this exercise.

STARTING POSITION

Stand with your feet separated the same width as your shoulders. Place your hands on your lower back, palms down.

EXERCISE

Lift your chest up towards the ceiling as you gently bend back over your hands as far as is comfortable. Make sure that your chin is facing forward.

Hold for three seconds.

Repeat three to five times.

This exercise should always be done after you have been sitting, bending or lifting.

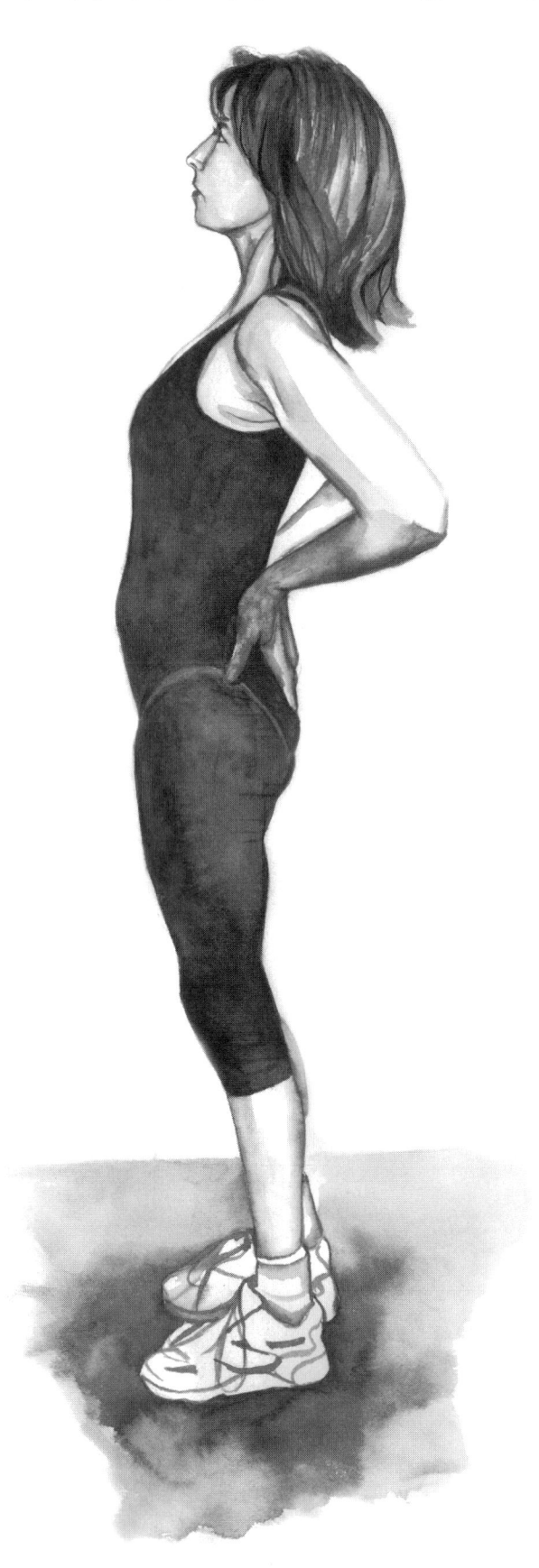

Stick 'Em Up
RESISTANCE EXERCISE

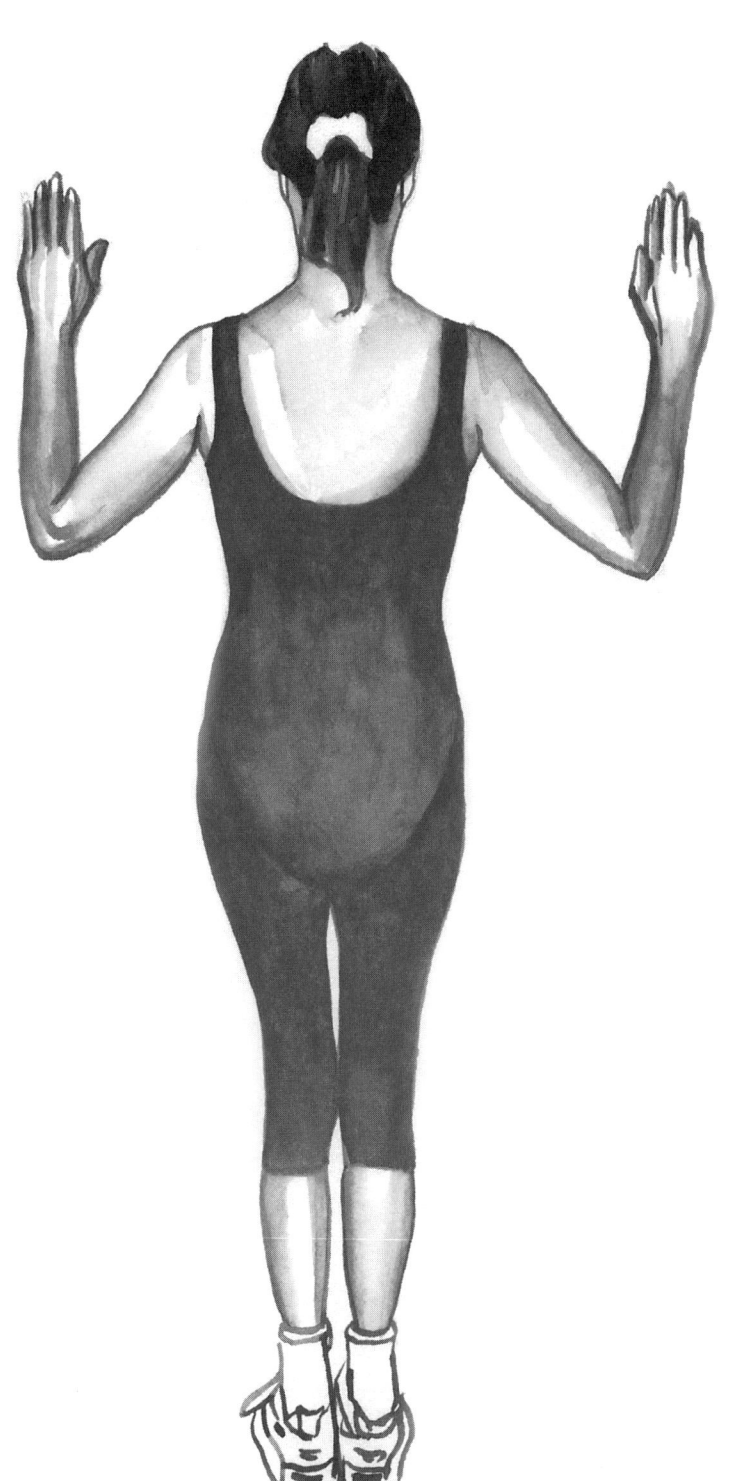

OBJECTIVE

To increase back strength.

STARTING POSITION

Sit or stand in a comfortable position.

If you are sitting, place your feet on the floor with your knees apart.

If you are standing, tighten your lower abdominal muscles and make sure your knees are soft (not locked).

Your back should be straight, but not rigid.

Place arms in a "W" position without hunching your shoulders.

EXERCISE

Bring your arms backwards to a comfortable position, while pinching your shoulder blades together.

Hold for three seconds and return to the starting position.

Work up to ten repetitions. When you can perform this exercise ten times without difficulty, add one-pound weights in each hand or around each wrist. You can gradually increase the amount of weight.

Balancing on One Leg
BALANCE EXERCISE

OBJECTIVE

To improve standing balance and muscle support.

STARTING POSITION

Stand in a comfortable, balanced position where there is a counter or sturdy chair to hold onto for support if needed.

Stand with your feet three to four inches apart.

Have your knees soft (not locked) and your toes facing forward.

EXERCISE

Tighten your lower abdominal muscles.

Lift your left knee to a comfortable position while you maintain the tightness in your lower abdominal muscles.

Hold for five to ten seconds. Think of your head and spine as lengthening upward while you perform this exercise.

Alternate legs and perform five to ten repetitions with each leg.

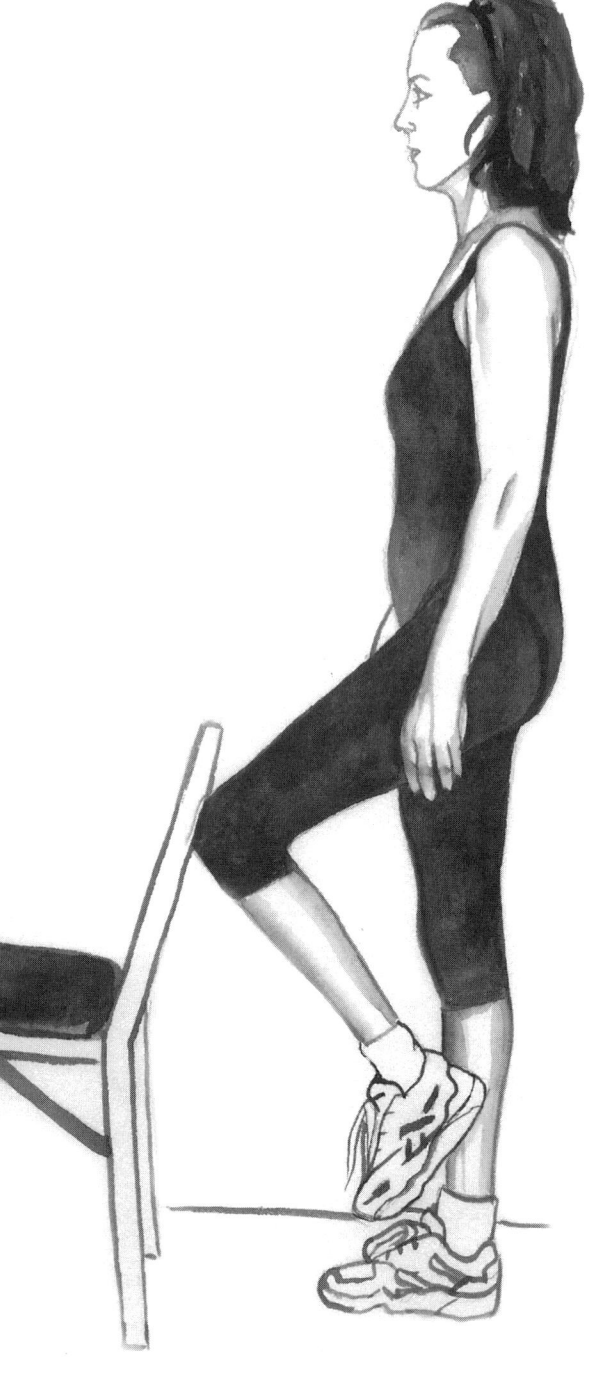

Standing Side Leg Lifts
RESISTANCE EXERCISE

OBJECTIVE

To strengthen your hip muscles and improve your balance.

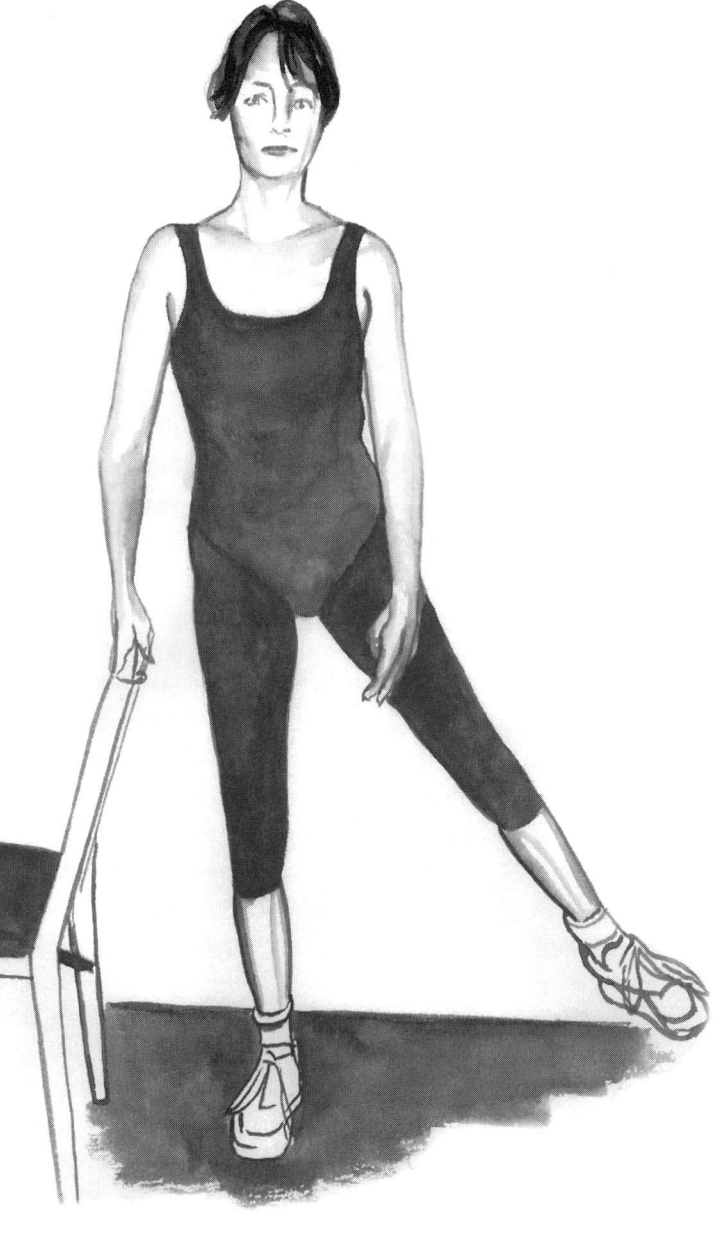

STARTING POSITION

Stand in a comfortable position with one hand holding a stable object.

Your knees and toes should be pointed forward.

Keep your body straight and tighten your lower abdominal muscles throughout the exercise.

Keep the knee of your standing leg slightly bent.

EXERCISE

Lift one leg out to the side, to a height that is comfortable.

Hold for three seconds.

Slowly lower your leg to the starting position.

Progress up to ten repetitions.

Repeat with the other leg, up to ten repetitions. When you can easily perform the exercise ten times, add a one-pound cuff weight to your ankle and repeat. You can gradually increase the amount of weight.

Standing Back Leg Lifts
RESISTANCE EXERCISE

OBJECTIVE

To strengthen your hip muscles and improve your balance.

STARTING POSITION

Stand in a comfortable position with both hands holding a stable object.

Your knees and toes should be pointed forward.

Keep your body straight and tighten your lower abdominal muscles throughout the exercise.

Keep the knee of your standing leg slightly bent.

EXERCISE

Bring one leg backwards to a comfortable level. Make sure not to bend forward.

Hold for three seconds.

Slowly lower your leg to the starting position.

Progress up to ten repetitions.

Repeat with the other leg, up to ten repetitions. When you can easily perform the exercise ten times, add a one-pound cuff weight to your ankle and repeat. You can gradually increase the amount of weight.

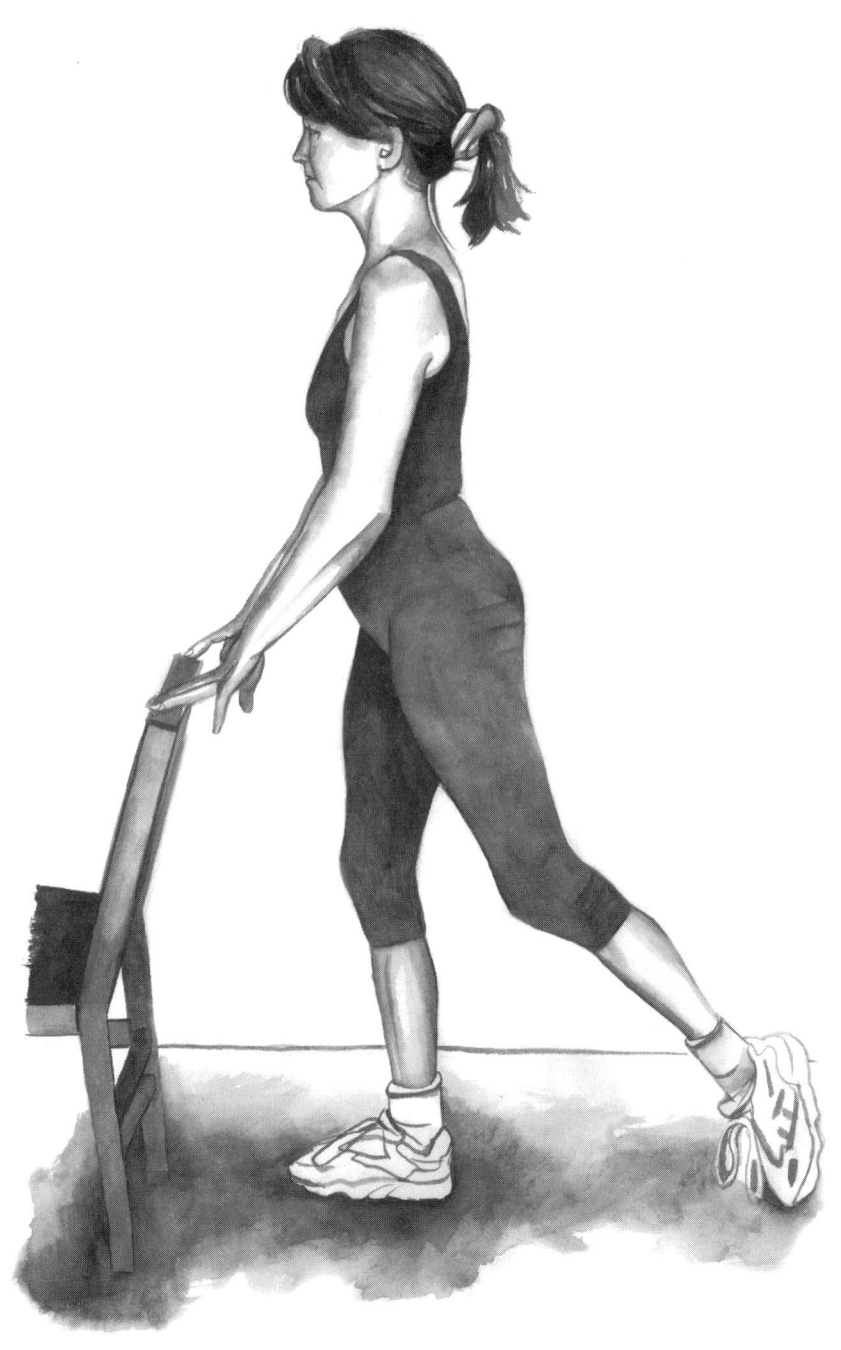

Wall-Slide

RESISTANCE EXERCISE

OBJECTIVE

To strengthen your thigh and knee muscles.

STARTING POSITION

Stand with your hips and shoulders against the wall.

Place your feet a few inches away from the wall. Keep your knees apart and feet forward.

Keep your spine lengthened.

EXERCISE

Gently tighten your lower abdominal muscles without losing your lower-back curve.

Bend your knees and slowly slide down the wall to a level that is comfortable and feels secure. Your buttocks should never go below your knees.

Hold this position for five to thirty seconds while maintaining your normal breathing pattern.

Slowly slide back up the wall.

This exercise should be performed only once each workout.

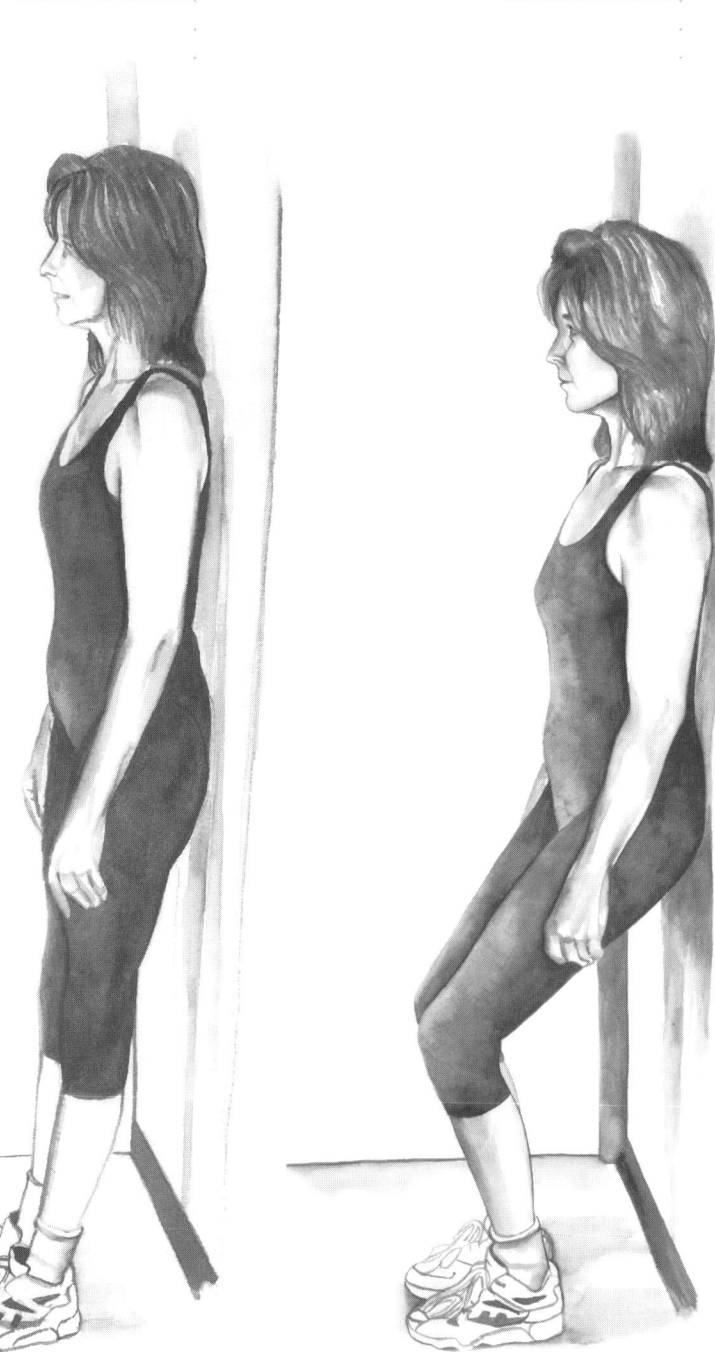

STEP ONE

STEP TWO

Straight Leg Raise

RESISTANCE EXERCISE

OBJECTIVE

To strengthen your thigh and abdominal muscles and stretch your hamstring muscles.

STARTING POSITION

Lie on your back with your right knee bent and left leg straight. You can use a small pillow or towel roll under your neck for comfort. You can also use a small folded towel under your lower back.

Tighten your abdominal muscles so that your back is flat against the floor or towel roll. Maintain this position throughout the exercise.

EXERCISE

Lift your left leg as high as is comfortable while keeping your left knee straight and left foot flexed up toward your head.

Hold for three seconds.

Slowly lower your leg, keeping your back flat against the floor.

Progress up to ten repetitions.

Repeat with the other leg, up to ten repetitions. Once you can easily perform this exercise, add one-pound cuff weights to your ankles and repeat. Gradually increase the amount of weight.

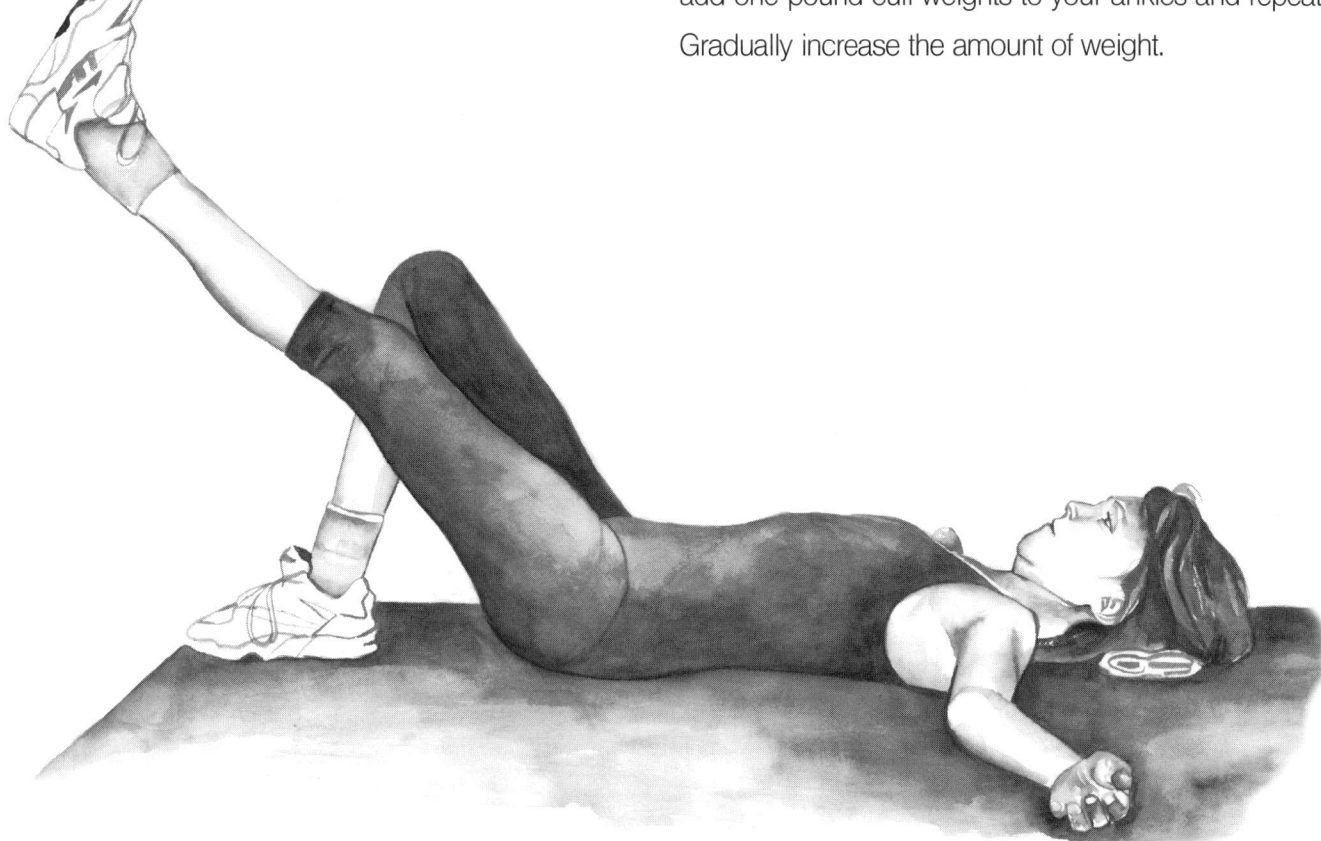

All-Fours Arm and Leg Lift

RESISTANCE EXERCISE

OBJECTIVE

To strengthen your back, hip, and wrist muscles. To improve your balance and coordination.

STARTING POSITION

Assume a hands-and-knees position with your head in a neutral position. Look at the floor.

Gently tighten your abdominal muscles while performing this exercise. Think of your back as a flat table and keep it stable throughout the exercise.

EXERCISE

Slowly raise your right arm off the floor and hold for three seconds. Repeat with your left arm.

Slowly raise your left leg off the floor and hold for three seconds. Repeat with your right leg.

Once you can do this, lift your right arm and left leg simultaneously and hold for three seconds. Make sure to keep your back flat.

Repeat with your left arm and right leg.

Alternate sides and perform up to ten repetitions on each side. Make sure to visualize your spine as lengthening throughout this exercise. When you can easily perform ten repetitions maintaining a stable position, you can add one-pound cuff weights to your wrists and ankles. You can gradually increase the amount of weight.

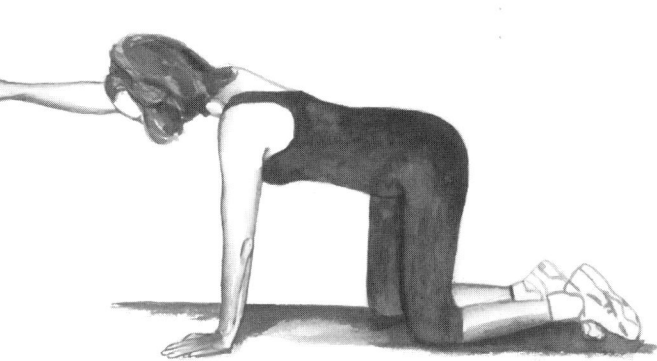
STEP ONE

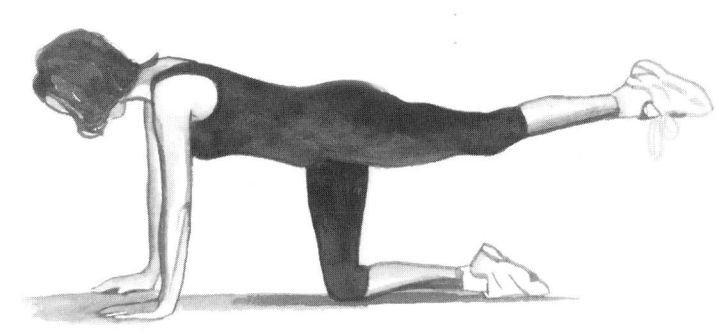
STEP TWO

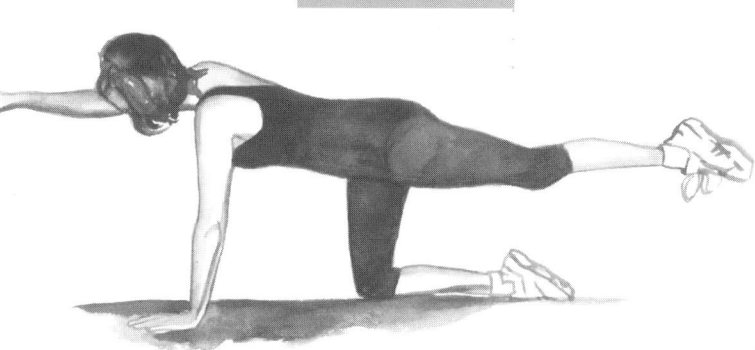
STEP THREE

Walking as an Exercise

Walking is an excellent weight-bearing exercise. It helps maintain and increase bone mass as well as strengthen back, leg and stomach muscles. Walking improves your cardiovascular fitness and increases the efficiency of your heart.

To achieve the maximum cardiovascular benefit for your age and fitness level, exercise at your target heart rate. Patients on certain heart or blood pressure medications should speak to their physicians about their target heart rates.

Your target heart rate is 60 to 80 percent of your maximum heart rate, depending on your fitness level. Your maximum heart rate is calculated by subtracting your age from 220. If you are just beginning, start at the 60 percent level. Contact your physician or physical therapist to determine your exercise range.

To monitor your heart rate, you need to check your pulse.

Place your index and middle fingers on the thumb side of your opposite wrist or the side of your throat next to your "Adam's apple."

Press lightly and feel your pulse.

Count the number of beats in ten seconds and multiply by six. This is your heart rate per minute. Throughout your walking program, you can monitor your pulse at timed intervals. Your goal is to reach your target heart rate.

If you experience dizziness, lightheadedness, chest pain or shortness of breath, discontinue exercising immediately and seek medical attention.

Before beginning any exercise program, speak with your physician regarding any restrictions!

TARGET HEART RATE

Age	Low intensity (60%)	Moderate intensity (70%)	High intensity (80%)
35	111	130	148
40	108	126	144
45	105	123	140
50	102	119	136
55	99	116	132
60	96	112	128
65	93	109	124
70	90	105	120
75	87	102	116
80	84	98	112
85	81	95	108

The Walking Program

BEFORE YOU WALK

- Make sure you are wearing walking or running shoes with good support and cushioning.

- Take your pulse for ten seconds and multiply by six for your resting heart rate.

- Do at least three minutes of slow walking or relaxed arm and leg movements before starting the flexibility exercises. These movements warm up the muscles and make it easier to stretch.

- Perform the heel cord, hip flexor, and hamstring stretches included on the next three pages before walking.

DURING YOUR WALK

- Lengthen your spine while you walk. Visualize your head floating up to the sky like a helium balloon.

- Make sure your buttocks' muscles are relaxed and your shoulders are moving freely.

- Warm up by walking at a slow-to-normal pace for the first five minutes.

- Increase your speed gradually until you are walking briskly.

- Take your ten-second pulse approximately five to ten minutes into your brisk walk to ensure you are working at the appropriate level (i.e., your target heart rate).

- Make sure you can talk comfortably while you are walking.

- Keep walking at a level that doesn't exhaust you and can be maintained for at least twenty minutes.

- Work up to a forty-five-minute walk.

- At the end of your walk, cool down with a five-minute slow walk. This safely lowers your pulse.

AFTER YOU WALK

- Repeat the heel cord, hip flexor, and hamstring stretches.

- Check your pulse and make sure it is lower than the level you reached during the brisk walk. If not, contact your physician before continuing with the program.

- Try to walk as often as possible. Walking three times a week is the minimum necessary to improve cardiovascular fitness and increase bone density. If you experience shortness of breath or chest pain while walking, stop immediately and contact your physician.

Heel Cord Stretch

WARM-UP EXERCISE

OBJECTIVE

To stretch your calf muscles.

STARTING POSITION

Stand with one leg forward and one leg back. Make sure that both knees are pointing forward.

Keep your back straight and place your hands on the wall at shoulder height.

EXERCISE

Bend your forward knee while keeping the heel of your back leg flat on the floor.

Bend until you feel a slight stretch in the calf of your back leg. Visualize your spine as lengthening upward as you stretch.

Hold for ten to twenty seconds.

Alternate legs and repeat two times with each leg.

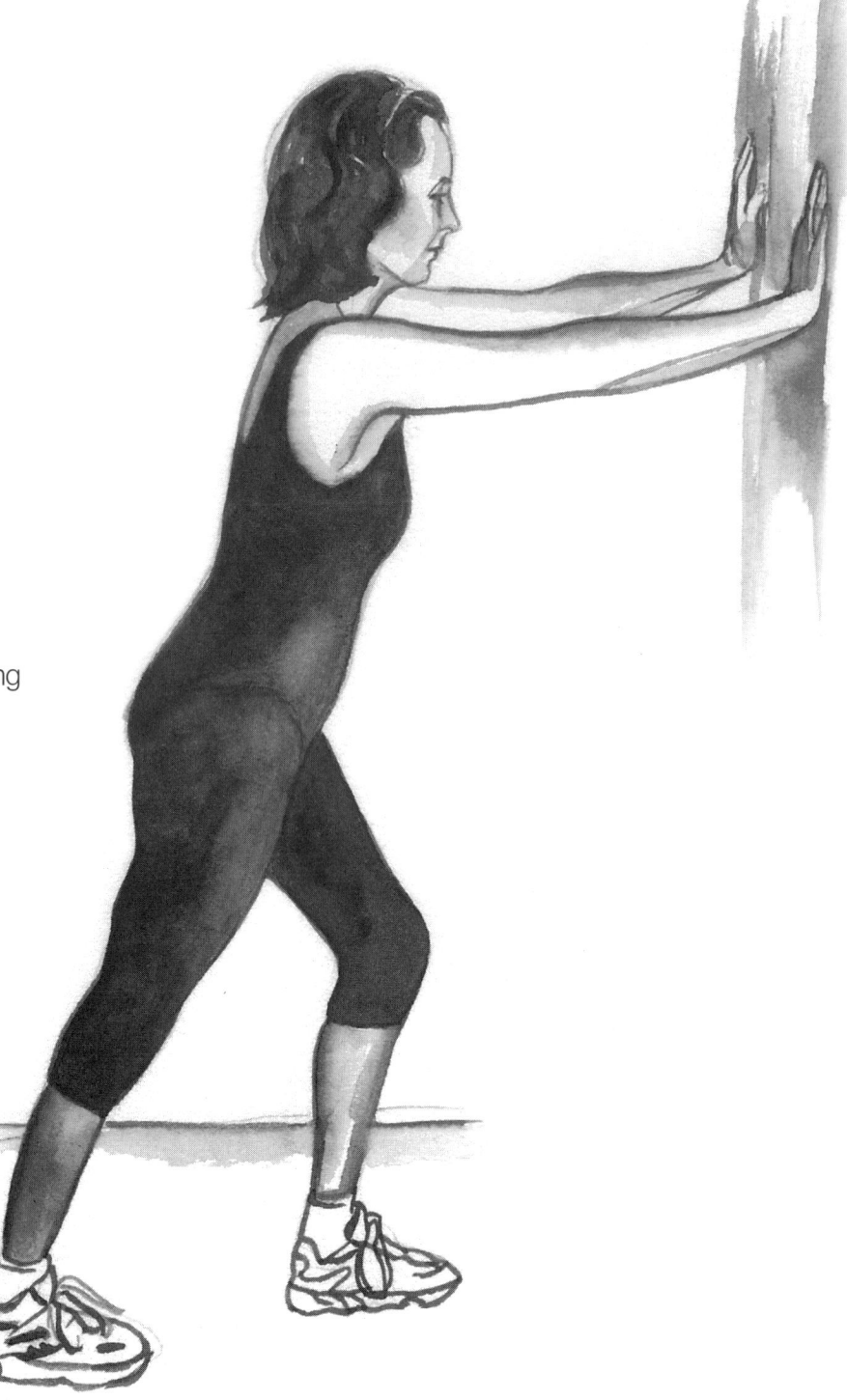

Hip Flexor Stretch
WARM-UP EXERCISE

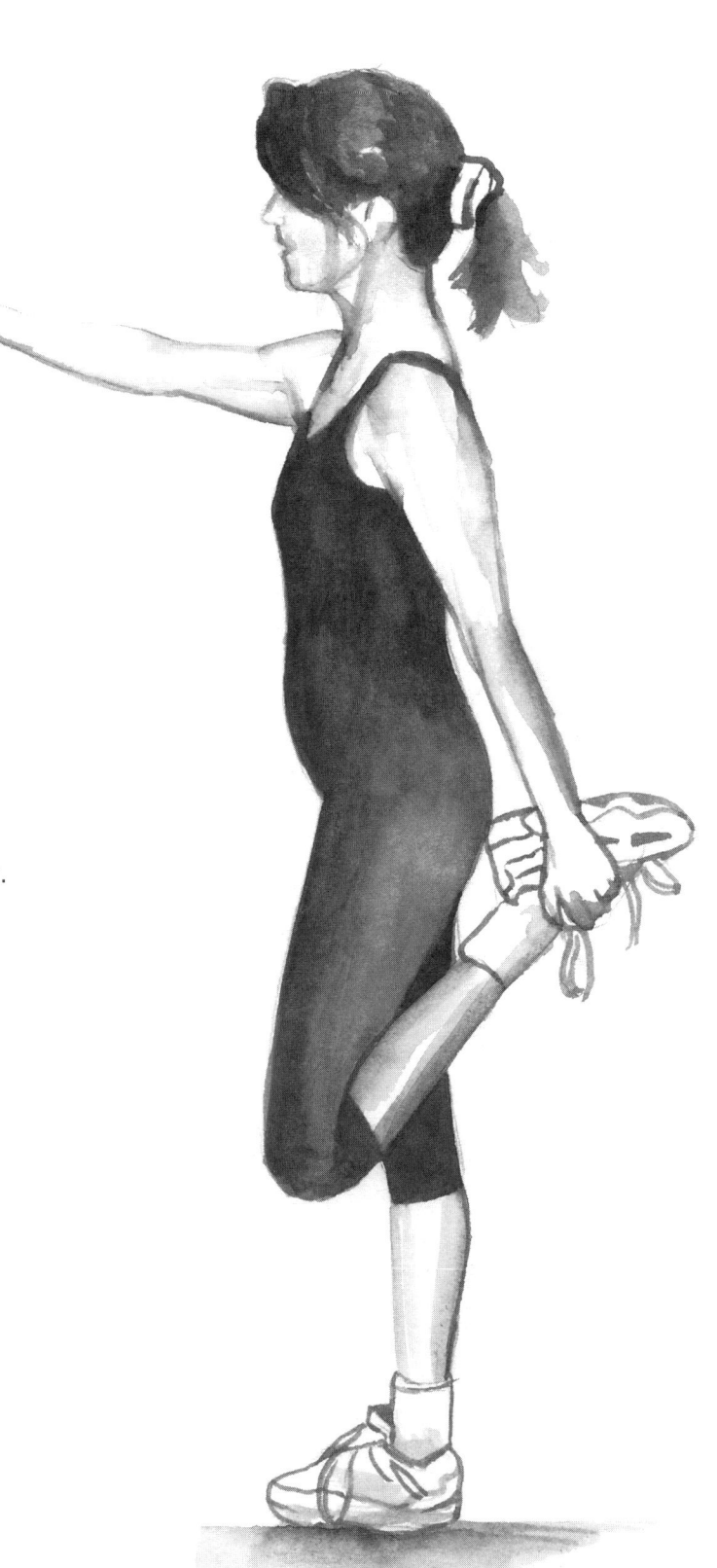

OBJECTIVE

To stretch the muscles on the front of your thighs.

STARTING POSITION

Stand in a comfortable, balanced position with your right hand holding onto the wall or a stable object for support. Keep your back straight and visualize your spine lengthening.

EXERCISE

Grasp above your left ankle with your left hand as you bend your left knee. Don't twist your back to reach your leg.

You should feel a slight stretch in the front of your left thigh.

Hold for ten to twenty seconds.

Alternate legs and repeat two times with each leg.

Standing Hamstring Stretch
WARM-UP EXERCISE

OBJECTIVE

To stretch your hamstring muscles.

STARTING POSITION

Stand in a comfortable position.

Hold onto a wall for balance.

EXERCISE

Place your right foot on a table or stool as high as is comfortable, keeping your right knee and back straight.

Keep your right foot at a right angle to your right leg.

You should feel a slight stretch in the back of your right knee. Otherwise, bend your left knee until you feel a slight stretch. Visualize your spine lengthening upward as you stretch.

Hold for ten to twenty seconds.

Alternate legs and repeat two times with each leg.

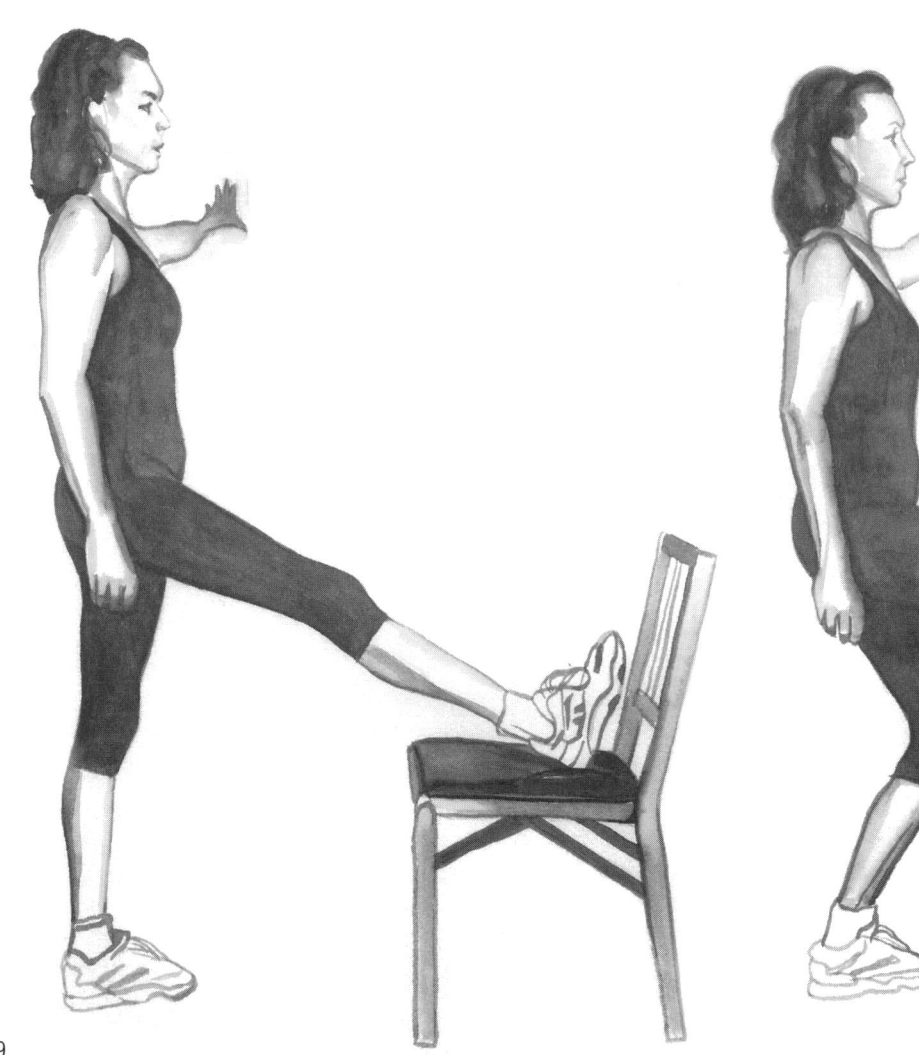
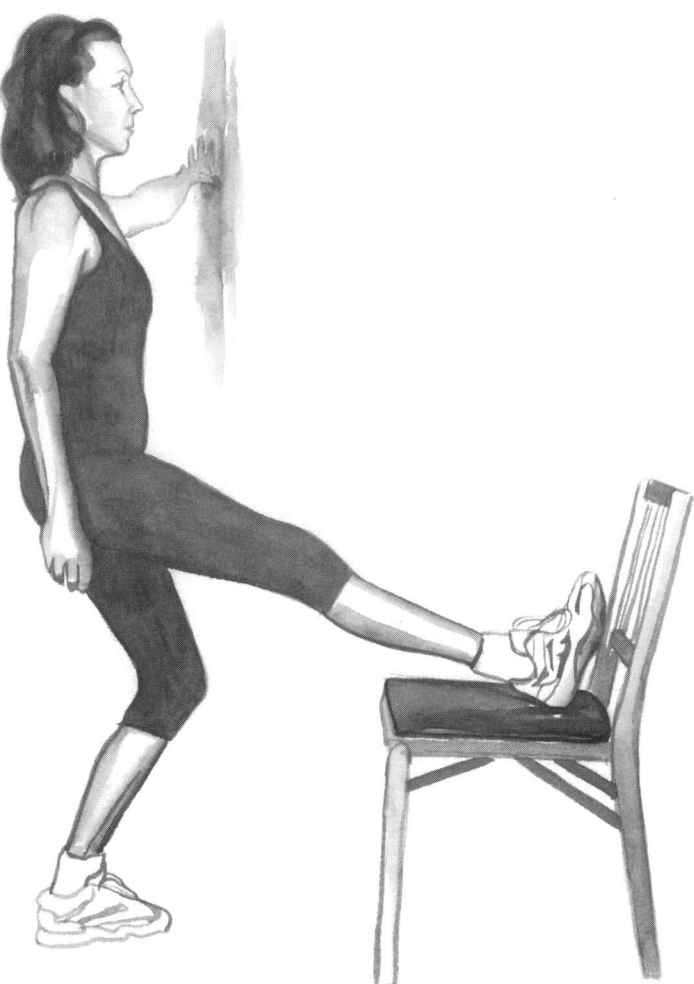

Suggested Exercise Program

DAILY EXERCISES

EXERCISE	TYPE	FREQUENCY	WEIGHTS
HEAD FORWARD AND UP	POSTURE	CONTINUOUS	NONE
SHOULDER STRETCH	POSTURE	3-5 TIMES A DAY	NONE
STANDING BACK-BEND	POSTURE	3-5 TIMES A DAY	NONE
BALANCING ON ONE LEG	BALANCE	2 TIMES A DAY	NONE

WEEKLY EXERCISES

EXERCISE	TYPE	FREQUENCY	WEIGHTS
STICK 'EM UP	RESISTANCE	2-3 TIMES A WEEK	YES
STANDING SIDE LEG LIFTS	RESISTANCE	2-3 TIMES A WEEK	YES
STANDING BACK LEG LIFTS	RESISTANCE	2-3 TIMES A WEEK	YES
WALL-SLIDE	RESISTANCE	2-3 TIMES A WEEK	NONE
STRAIGHT LEG RAISE	RESISTANCE	2-3 TIMES A WEEK	YES
ALL-FOURS ARM AND LEG LIFT	RESISTANCE	2-3 TIMES A WEEK	YES
THE WALKING PROGRAM	WEIGHT BEARING	3-7 TIMES A WEEK	NONE

Activities of Daily Living

This exercise program is just one important step in taking charge of your health. Proper nutrition and routine visits to your physician are other vital ingredients to a healthy life. One area of our life is often overlooked. It is what we do each day. We refer to this concept as "Activities of Daily Living."

While exercising, we focus on posture and strength. But what about the rest of the day? Do we bend or lift properly? Even people who exercise regularly are susceptible to household injuries.

To help prevent needless injuries, I have provided additional suggestions for safely performing some common tasks.

Please practice these instructions and hints with the same care you apply to your regular exercises.

Sitting with Support

Many people in our society sit in a slumped position that rounds the lower back. This posture puts forceful pressure on the lower back, upper back, head and neck regions and can lead to injury.

TECHNIQUE

When sitting, your feet should be flat on the floor. Ideally, you should have a chair that is adjustable for height. If not, a footrest can be used under your feet.

Your normal lower back curve should be supported by the chair. To do this, the chair back should curve slightly forward. This support is necessary to avoid slumping. If your chair does not have a low back support, you can place a lumbar roll or rolled towel in the small of your lower back for support.

It is very important to get up frequently from sitting — at least once an hour. Remember to sit with your spine lengthened, with your head floating up, and your shoulders wide. Good sitting habits are more important than chair design.

WHEN DRIVING

The same principles hold true when you are driving. Some cars have a lumbar support in the seat which you should adjust to support your lower back curve. You can also use a towel roll or a portable lumbar roll if your car seat does not give you adequate back support.

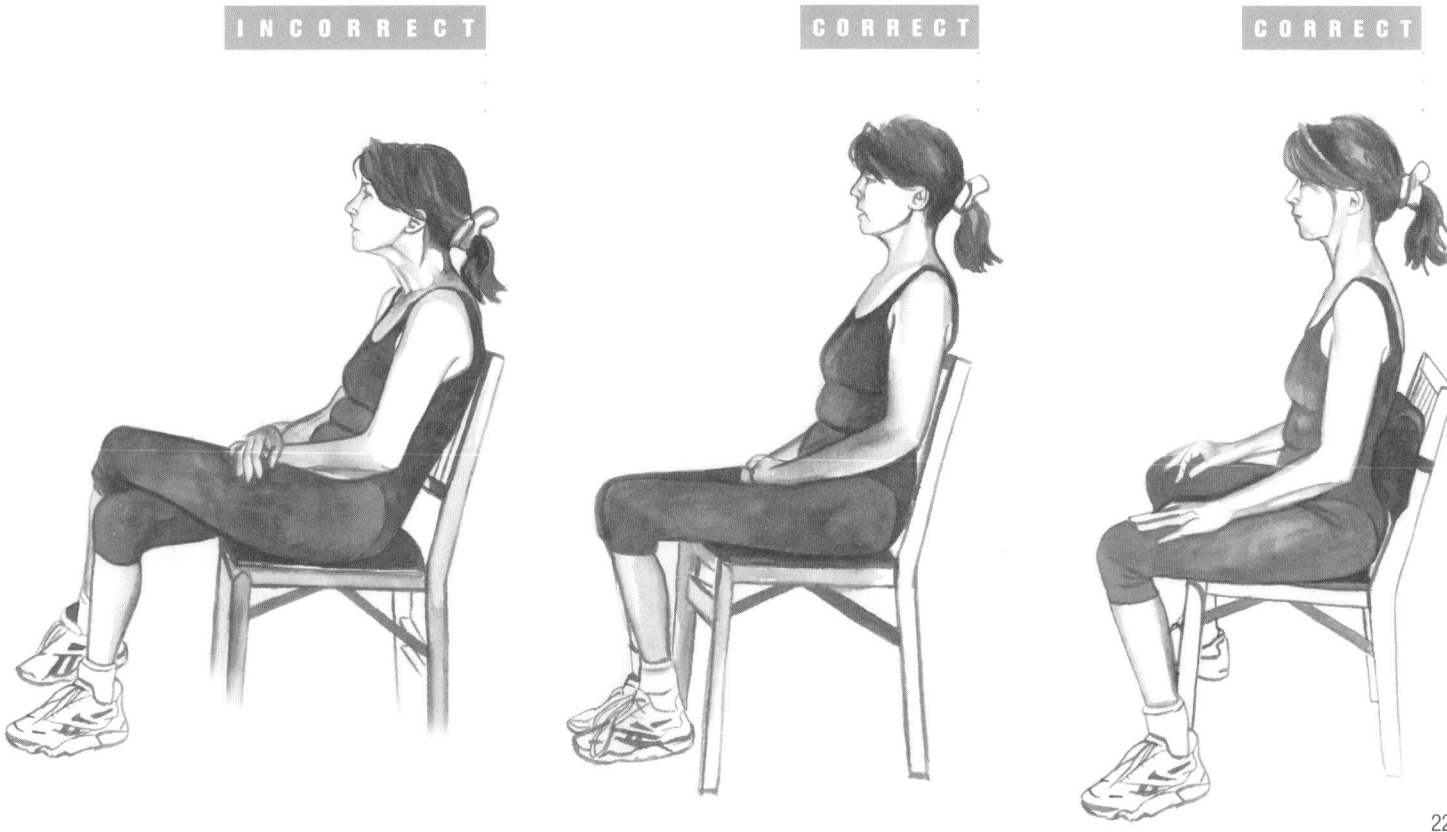

INCORRECT   CORRECT   CORRECT

Sitting without Support

There are times when you cannot rely on the chair back for support. It is important to sit in a comfortable, balanced position. Avoid sitting with your back rounded.

TECHNIQUE

Sit close to the front of a firm chair with your knees apart. To find a good sitting position, place your hands under your buttocks and feel for the two bony lumps (sit bones). When you slump, the sit bones move forward. If you arch your back too much, then the sit bones elevate off the chair. When you are sitting properly, the sit bones should be resting directly into your hands.

Placing a small rolled towel under your buttocks can tilt your pelvis forward and help prevent slumped sitting. Remember to sit with your spine lengthened and your shoulders wide.

Sitting without any support may become tiring and should be alternated with other sitting postures.

It is very important to get up frequently from sitting — at least once an hour.

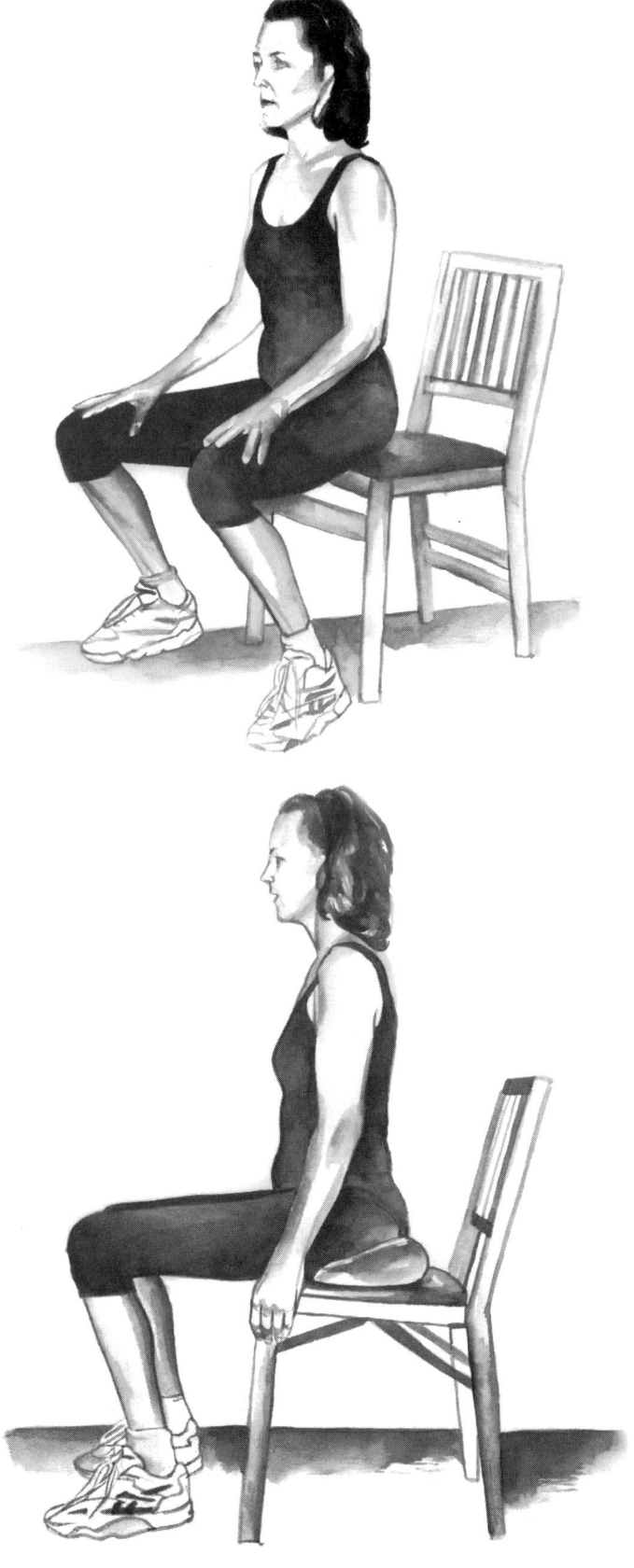

Bending from the Hips

It is important that you bend from the hips and not the waist. The hips are located deep in the folds where your legs join your trunk. It is helpful to visualize your body as being divided into an upper and lower half, with the hips being the dividing line. This is where your movement should take place.

TECHNIQUE

Place your hands on your stomach and back to make sure that you are keeping your trunk straight. Do not bend from the waist.

Lead with your head and chest, and bend forward with the movement occurring at the hips and knees.

Maintain your normal low back curve.

This type of bending can be used to perform many daily activities (making a bed, loading the dishwasher, brushing your teeth, etc.) Bending from the hip is also an effective method of getting in and out of a chair.

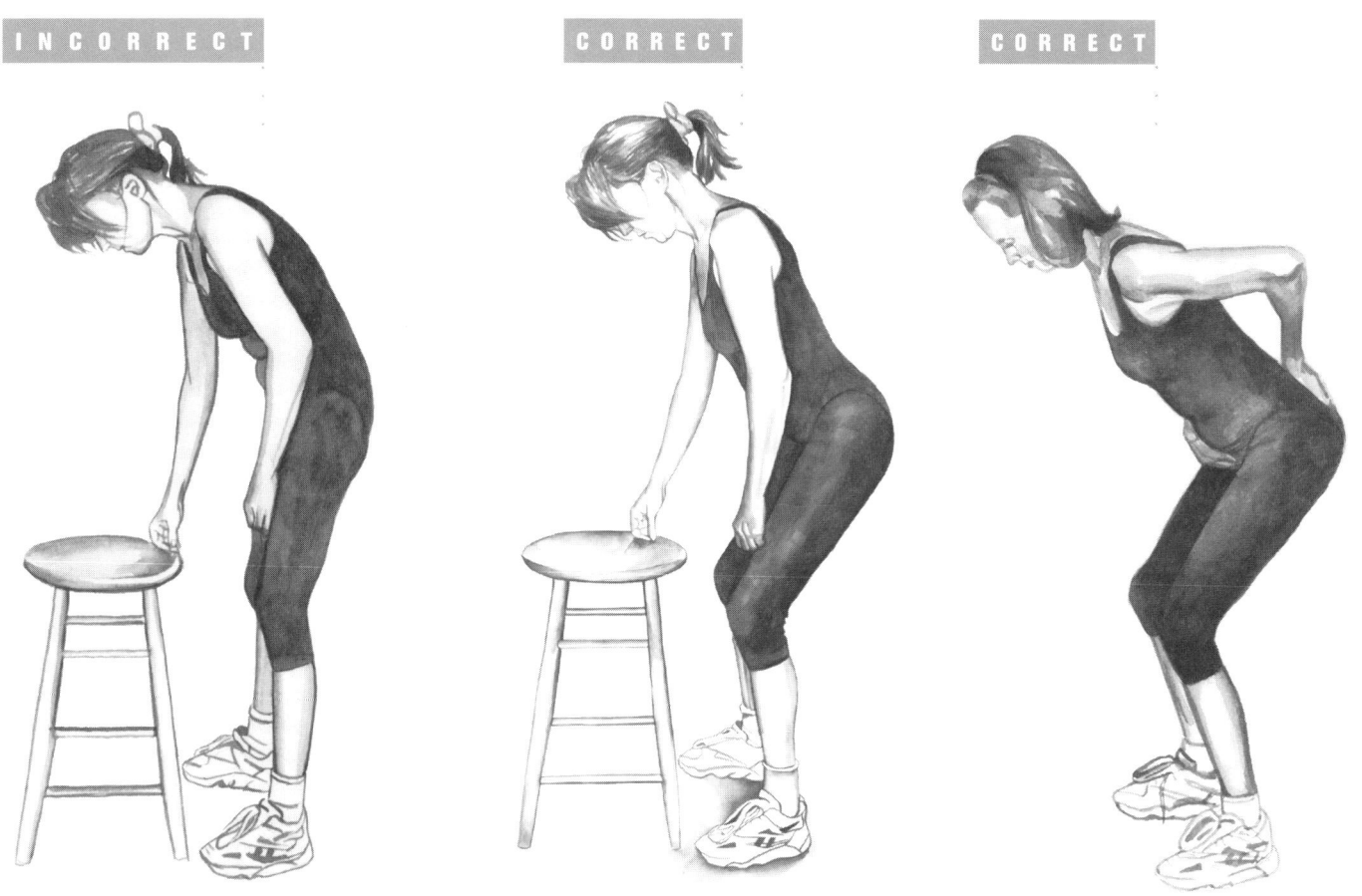

INCORRECT   CORRECT   CORRECT

Coughing or Sneezing

The sudden force of a cough or sneeze can cause your spine to bend forward suddenly. This natural event can lead to injuries of the spine and vertebral fractures. It is very important to stabilize your back in anticipation of a cough or sneeze.

TECHNIQUES

- You can place one hand in the small of your lower back to help you stand erect during the cough or sneeze.

- Bend your knees, bend your hips, keep your back lengthened, and place one hand on your thigh. This will help stabilize your back and keep it in alignment. Practice both of these methods so that you are prepared when you need to sneeze or cough.

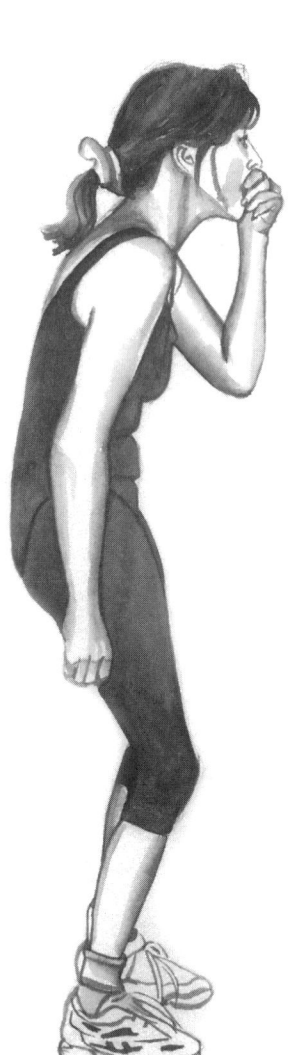

INCORRECT

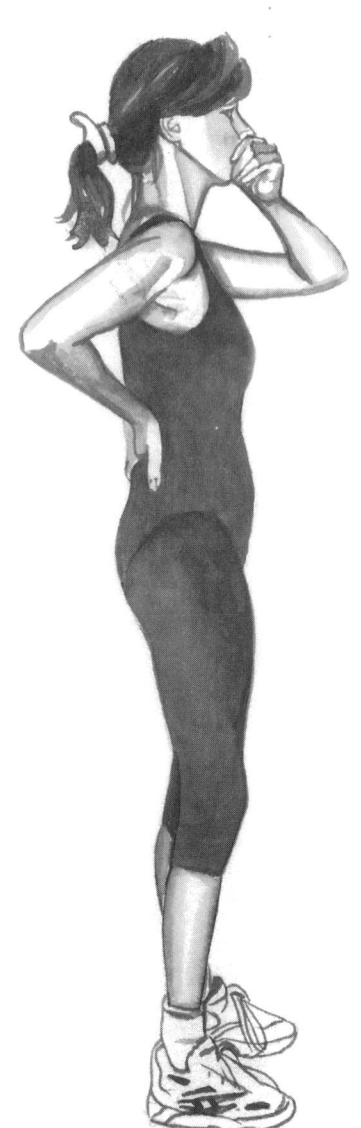

CORRECT

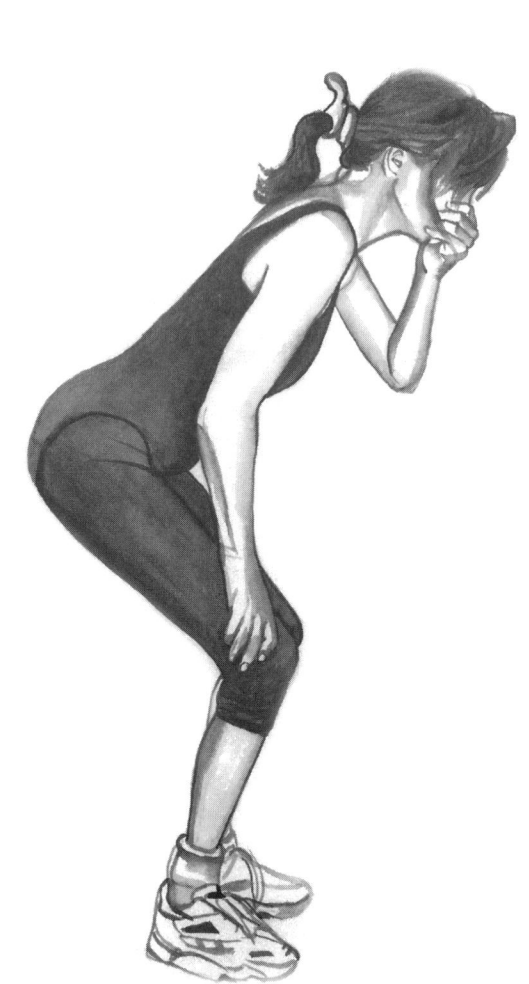

CORRECT

Vacuuming, Mopping, Raking

For all daily activities, it is important to avoid bending forward from the waist. Use your hips and knees to bend. Maintain the arch in your low back during daily activities. Avoid twisting and especially the combination of forward bending and twisting. It is always better to push rather than pull an object if you have the choice.

TECHNIQUE

Use the momentum and power of your legs to perform the motion.

If you are moving an object forward and backwards – such as a vacuum – have one leg in front of the other, knees bent, and rock from foot to foot while maintaining your spine in a lengthened position.

If you are moving an object – such as a mop – sideways, rock from leg to leg sideways, knees bent, while maintaining your spine in a lengthened position.

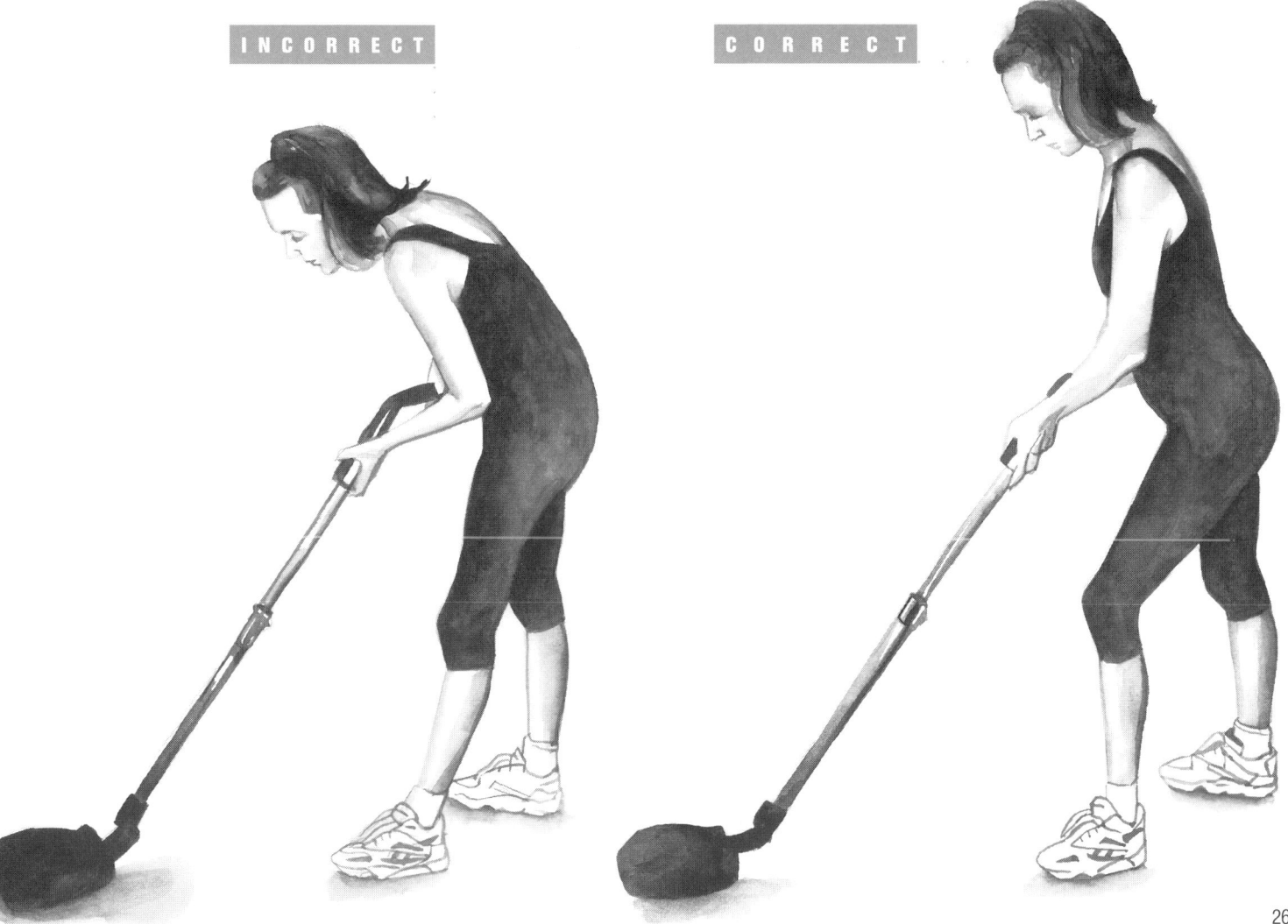

INCORRECT

CORRECT

To Your Health!

Congratulations on completing this exercise guide. It offers you a beginning to your lifelong journey to good health. Not only will it help reduce your risk or degree of osteoporosis, but it will improve your overall fitness and quality of life.

The principles discussed in this guide can be applied to a variety of exercises and daily activities. Be your own fitness expert. When you are aware of safe body movements, you can avoid needless injuries. If you have any questions or need further guidance, contact a physical therapist or physician.

For more information, visit
www.workfitonline.com

I welcome your comments. You can reach me by e-mail.
Margie@workfitonline.com

Following are several other resources which complement this book.

American Physical Therapy Association
1111 North Fairfax Street
Alexandria, VA 22314-1488
phone: **800-999-2782**

National Osteoporosis Foundation
1150 17th Street
Suite 500
Washington, DC 20036-4603
phone: **202-223-2226**

Back Trouble: A New Approach to Prevention and Recovery
by D. Caplan
Triad Publishing Company
Gainesville, FL, 1987